*A*ctions,

*B*alance,
and

*C*aring

for TBI

A guide for Family Members dealing with a Loved One's Traumatic Brain Injury

Dedication

There were many family members, friends, and acquaintances that prayed for and offered support to my husband and me. Their care and concern will always be special to us both. However, there are four individuals who made this book possible: my husband Jim for having the courage to continue fighting to regain himself, Dr. Toms (Geisinger) who gave Jim his life, Susan - Jim's BlueCross/BlueShield Case manager who was always a phone call away and who encouraged me to write this when the time was right, and my best friend Sue who gave me the courage to "just do it".

My husband suffered a Traumatic Brain Injury on September 24, 2011. He was in a very critical state. He had to have his left side skull plate removed and his brain swelled three centimeters. The doctors did not expect him to make it through the first night and he remained in a coma for over a week. His journey included a total of two months in the Adult Intensive Care Unit and then an Acute Care Hospital, followed by an additional two months in a rehabilitation center. He returned home January 6th, still without his skull plate. That was replaced January 19th, 2012.

Although I read many books and articles on the subject, there was much more that I learned through trial and error. I was fortunate that my years of teaching students with learning differences enabled me to use that experience to develop ways of helping my husband improve to a level of "near normalcy" one year later. My goal for writing this is to share some lessons that I learned with you – the care giver of a loved one who has been diagnosed with a Traumatic Brain Injury. I have included blank pages at the end of each section for you to make "reminder" notes as you use this handbook.

After the shock of hearing the severity of the injury wears off and you have time to think, there are many things that you should keep in mind. What follows is a list of the "actions" that I found useful.

While your loved one is in the ICU and/or Acute Care Ward:

1. Find out when the doctors are making their rounds and be in the room while they are reviewing his/her chart. Get to know the physician assistant. That is the person who will have the time and information to answer your question

2. Get caller ID so that you can -honestly- screen your calls and keep track of calls missed

3. Keep a small notebook, with an attached pen, to write down names and numbers of health care providers, support people, and anyone else that you don't usually have contact with by telephone.

4. Read...read...read. There are many books and internet sites on the subject. You don't need to get technical, just have awareness.

5. While your loved one is in the hospital, it isn't necessary to spend the entire day by his/her side. For an example, I went in the morning to be there when the doctors made their rounds and then stayed until lunch and returned to work in the afternoon. I was able then to use only $\frac{1}{2}$ sick days and I could focus on something other than my husband's injury.

6. If your insurance provider incorporates a Case Manager Program and you are contacted by one, accept that help. She will be a great source of information and guidance.

7. If your loved one has been employed, use the internet and download the paperwork for Social Security Disability Income.

(http://www.ssa.gov/pgm/disability.htm) Start it

while the person is in the hospital as you will need reports from the doctors. If your loved one was seriously injured that may include the initial emergency room, the intensive care unit, acute care unit, and the rehabilitation center's doctors. It will be much easier to get the forms completed while the person is a patient than to try to backtrack later.

8. Contact your loved one's place of employment Human Resource office. Some employers have an insurance program that provides short term wage coverage. There will be forms that the doctor will need to complete.

9. Keep a log :

   a. It will give you something to focus on and stay organized

b. It will assist your loved one with closing the gap of the time missed while in the hospital and rehabilitation center.

10. While your loved one is in the acute care center, start investigating rehabilitation centers that work with head injuries. If you wait, you may have only a week to decide and therefore additional stress for you. Do not hesitate to ask his/her physician for their recommendations.

    (http://www.headinjury.com/rehabfacility.htm)

11. Visit a lawyer who specializes in health issues. Usually this would be an attorney who focuses on elder law. If this is your spouse, you will want to make sure that paperwork is in order to protect your assets. You should also set up a trust in case you are unable to care for the person. If you do

not have Power of Attorney, get one written as soon as your spouse is able to understand and sign. Your attorney will assist with this.

12. Take photos of where the person worked and of their co-workers (or school, teachers, friends), along with family members, and any particular interests that the person may have (sports, hobbies, etc). Print them as 5x7s and write names, dates, etc on the back. Place them in the room so that he/she can see them. Also, the nurses and Speech Therapists can use them to assist your loved one with recall and language skills. If there is a particular type of music that your loved one usually listened to, buy an inexpensive CD player and CDs for the staff to play for him/her in the room.

13. If the person is a male and usually has facial hair, make sure to let the staff know. My husband of 34 years always had a beard and moustache, imagine my horror when I came to visit and it was all gone! The nurse's aide quickly made a large "Do Not Shave" sign and placed it over his bed.

Your Notes - such as the time the doctors make their rounds, the case manager's name and phone number, etc.

While the person is at a Rehabilitation Center

14. When you visit your loved one, you may notice that he/she will be very angry toward you. This both devastated and irritated me. How could he be so mean to me? The staff there explained that this is normal and that the person would soon stop and even not remember that they were nasty. They are not aware of where they are and why. Therefore, they will be angry with their closest loved one; parent, child, or spouse. As hard as it will be on you, keep in mind that this is a normal phase and it too such pass.

15. Surround yourself with people. You will need time to enjoy yourself, to just forget for awhile your loved one and to focus on what makes you happy. You may feel guilty, don't! My family and friends kept me sane and gave me strength to carry on.

16. Join a support group for Brain Injury if there is one local and it fits into your schedule.

17.   If your loved one is school age- contact the local Intermediate Unit or the district's Director of Special Education. You want to locate a program such as Brain Steps or something similar. Also once the student returns to school, he or she will be eligible for a 504 (American with Disabilities Act) or perhaps an Individualized Educational Plan, depending on the level of accommodations and adaptations necessary for him/her to access the curriculum.

18. Keep three small binders

   a. One for copies of doctors' reports and visits (after your loved one comes home). You should take this with you when you visit the doctors.

b. Another for all bills paid and expenses. This will make it much easier when you file your end of year taxes.

c. The third one for miscellaneous notices and information such as the rehabilitation centers or home health care providers. Also, if the person is school age, you would keep any 504 Plan or Individualized Educational Plans paperwork in this notebook.

19. Purchase adult size disposable underpants for the staff to use there. First, they are more appropriate than the institutional kind and secondly, these will be easier for the person to use as they begin their journey to independence.

20 Before your loved one is scheduled to leave the rehabilitation center, check to see if your state has a

Brain Injury Program. Find out what the requirements are and which agencies, in your area, are available to provide support.

21. Also, before returning home, have the Rehabilitation's Case Manager complete forms for a Handicap Parking placard.

Your Notes – such as the case manager's, doctor's, and therapists' names and phone numbers and agencies' contacts

When the loved one comes home:

22. Before your loved one returns home, have someone - visiting nurses or Center for Independent Living - visit your home to make sure that it is a safe environment. If you are concerned that your family member may leave the home while you are busy, hardware stores sell a very inexpensive doorstopper that when the door is opened a loud alarm is emitted.

23. You may notice that they are tired, easily agitated, and have a low frustration level. This is normal. Although swearing tends to be normal, do not tolerate it. Work on getting them to understand that yelling and cursing is not acceptable behavior. My husband developed a habit of screaming and swearing at me. I used card stock and printed out two signs with an unhappy face along with the

words "Stop Yelling at ME!" One for inside the house and another I kept next to my driver's seat in the car.

24. Help your loved one to remember things by using index cards and writing names and other important information down. My husband became used to this and began to write his own notes down when he found certain things difficult to remember (such as our grandson's names).

25. Be aware that the person has lost time. For an example: my husband was injured in September while football was on TV. He came home in January – no football. He informed our son that the "new" TV provider that I had didn't carry football. He had been spending hours looking for it.

26. For tasks around the house- here are two suggestions that will make life easier for you and the person with the TBI:

    a. Do task analyses - simply stop and take notice of the various individual steps that you follow when doing a particular "daily" activity. EX: making coffee.

        i. Get filter

        ii. Put filter in holder

        iii. Add 5 scoops (or whatever you use)

        iv. Place filter in holder

        v. Turn on facet

        vi. Fill container to line

        vii. Pour water into coffee maker

        viii. Replace container

        ix. Turn on machine

b. Make cards with the step by step directions on it – concise, keep the wording down. Tape the cards where they can be seen. I knew when my husband no longer required the cue cards- they went missing!

27. Depending on where the injury occurred – most individuals will respond quicker to visual cues in place of telling them. For most part their short term memory is a mess and they just won't remember!

The microwave completely baffled my husband. We posted step by step directions AND covered any button that wasn't going to be used.

28. Most head injuries will result in some aphasia. Either Receptive (they can hear but it doesn't make sense or it makes sense to them, but it isn't what was said to them) or Expressive – what they say makes

sense to them but not to you. For an example: after having his skull plate replaced he no longer needed his protective helmet. One day he asked me "Where is my hat for the rollers?" I thought about it and then looked at him – he was at the bottom of the stairs- so what he really was asking was where was his helmet for the steps. Six months later he asked me if I knew where his "toe rings where". Now that stumped me (trust me, my 60 year old husband would not wear toe rings!) until I looked down and saw that he was barefoot. He wanted to know where his flip flops where. When figuring out the "goofy" things that they may utter (and it will be goofy- keep a sense of humor) be aware it makes total sense to them and they may be frustrated that you don't respond right away. When talking with them be aware of the surroundings and what is occurring. You will be surprised how quickly you will then be able to figure it out.

29. To deal with Receptive Aphasia be sure that you speak normally; not quickly or too many sentences or thoughts strung together. The person needs time to process each concept. This is harder that it sounds. Think of how you speak to a toddler when you want them to do something: one step at a time.

30. Explain to the person what Aphasia is. I have read it likened to a filing cabinet that has been toppled and all the files are strewn about. Try to find an analogy that the person would understand. Such as a high school student would be told that his back pack fell and all the papers, books, pencils, etc came out and were quickly jammed back into the back pack. All the

tools and information is in there - just not in the folders or compartments where they belong. My husband worked on electrical panels, so I told him it was like a panel with faulty wiring and connections. The wires and connectors are present they just aren't hooked p properly.

31. Find crossword puzzles developed for elementary level children. This is a great activity to strengthen the person's language skills. Don't bother with the crossword books that are labeled "Easy or Very Easy". There is too much information on one page and will only become frustrating.

32. Have your loved one give you directions to complete tasks or when you are driving them to places they went to before the accident.

33. Do not coddle the person. Allow him/her to gain as much independence as possible. There may be setbacks but by keeping high expectations you will assist the person with regaining much more than may have been expected.

34. Find simple projects for him or the two of you to complete. It will give him/her a sense of normalcy and help the two of you to focus on something other than their limitations. My husband decided that our two car garage needed painted. So the two of us hand scraped and painted it over a span of two weeks. It sounded overwhelming, but it was great "medicine" for both of us. We had fun, he felt productive, and we had a common area to focus on. This activity also gave him the confidence to move on to projects that he

could complete on his own such as scraping and painting the back porch.

35. Some TBI patients make up stories. They are not aware that they had a brain injury and will invent explanations. My husband's rehabilitation center's psychologist called it "fabrication speech". This persisted after he returned home. Be consistent when "correcting" his/her perception of events and people. I was told of a man who took six years before being totally aware of his brain injury! Thankfully, my husband could explain his language difficulty within ten months. Although there are times he needs to be reminded.

36. You may notice that your loved one will "fixate" on things. This fixation may seem insignificant to you and may even become annoying. As long as it is not "life

threatening", just roll with it. They may soon find something new to fixate on.

37. Another thing that I noticed and didn't recall reading about is that as my husband's brain repaired itself, he appeared to go through "developmental phases". In the beginning everything was ALL about him; his needs, wants, and interests. Then his actions and comments reminded me of a three year old fighting for independence. It was actually humorous when months later I noticed that when talking to him it was if I was talking with a teenager: he would roll his eyes, make faces, and even argue for the sake of arguing. I often remarked that I hoped he would not go through a mid-life crisis as I was too old for that!

38. IMPORTANT: find a time and place where you can have "me time". This may be playing games on the

computer, curled up in the corner with a good book, taking walks, or meeting friends for coffee. This is time AWAY from the person with TBI, as the person many times becomes very needy on the caregiver. Let your loved one know that you need this time to stay rejuvenated. After spending all day with my husband, he now knows that by 9:00 pm on week nights I will be a basement dweller watching my television shows.

Dealing with others and outside agencies

39. As soon as he was able, I took my husband to functions and places where he could interact with other adults. We are lucky; we belong to numerous social organizations. At first, I tended to "run interference", until I realized that the people knew he had an accident and that they were able to converse

with him without my "interpreting". That was a wise move as it forced Jim to "find" the correct words so others would understand him.

40. If a recommendation is made to have a neuropsychological evaluation completed, I would recommend that you contact the psychologist's office to determine if they are experienced in dealing with TBI. Secondly, I would also recommend that your loved one's hearing is assessed first. In my husband's experience, we were not aware of a total hearing loss in his right ear. That loss, along with the Aphasia, clearly interfered with some of the validity of the test results. Also, individuals with TBI have a short attention span. The evaluation that is given can take up to five or more hours. I would highly suggest that you find a nearby neuropsychologist so that the test

can be administered over several days. I drove my husband two hours away. He was tested from 8:00 am until noon and then from 1:00 until 5:00 pm. The report that I received was not very encouraging. In hindsight, it was definitely not in Jim's best interest to have a two hour drive and then an all day evaluation.

41. The most important thing to keep in mind is that you KNOW your loved one; their likes, dislikes, attitude, and personality. You will deal with many individuals who are professionals in the medical and therapeutical world. You may be tempted to remain timid and allow their expertise to "overwhelm" you. Don't! You are your loved one's best advocate and spokesperson. You have an expertise in that person. It is that expertise that will assist your loved one with improving day-by-day.

Medication

42. First write every medication down; the dosage and when taken.

43. Purchase a daily pill container. You will probably need one with both AM and PM holders. You may also want to purchase a pill splitter. Many medications for seizures are gradually increased.

44. As soon as you determine that your loved one can, have him manage his pills. Write down the name and appearance of the pills; one list for Morning and one for Evening.

45. Be aware that some medications can have side effects that are not listed on the informational packet. Look up all medications on the internet to learn about them as much as possible. Unfortunately,

one of my husband's seizure medications made him lactose intolerant. This was not a stated side effect, but something I discovered when investigating his symptoms of irritable bowels. Removing excess dairy products and including OTC probiotic tablets solved that issue. Don't be afraid to take matters into your own hands, just let the doctor know what you discovered.

46. As my husband became more independent, such as taking the bus to exercise classes at the YMCA, I purchased two items from the local drugstore. One was a Medical ID bracelet and another was an ICE Medical Card (www.medicalid.com) that he carries in his wallet. Within the ID bracelet there is a note directing the medical staff to the ICE card in his wallet. The ICE card contains a thumb drive that when

inserted into a computer opens up to an Excel spread sheet with taps for personal information, physicians' names, prescriptions, and medical history. This gives me a peace of mind that if he was to have a seizure while I am not with him, pertinent information is available immediately for the medical staff attending to him.

Every Traumatic Brain Injury is unique to itself, as every human is unique unto his or herself. Don't be afraid to try "thinking outside the box" to assist your loved one with their recovery. It has been 12 months since my husband was injured. Unfortunately, his seizures started 7 months after the injury and we are working on finding the right medicine and dosage. However, other then his quirky communication skills and fixations on some things, many people have remarked that one would never known that one year ago he wasn't expected to live . It has been a struggle – sometimes more for the caregiver than for the patient, but humor, diligence, and optimism can help pave the way to an as normal a recovery as possible.

Things you want to remember:

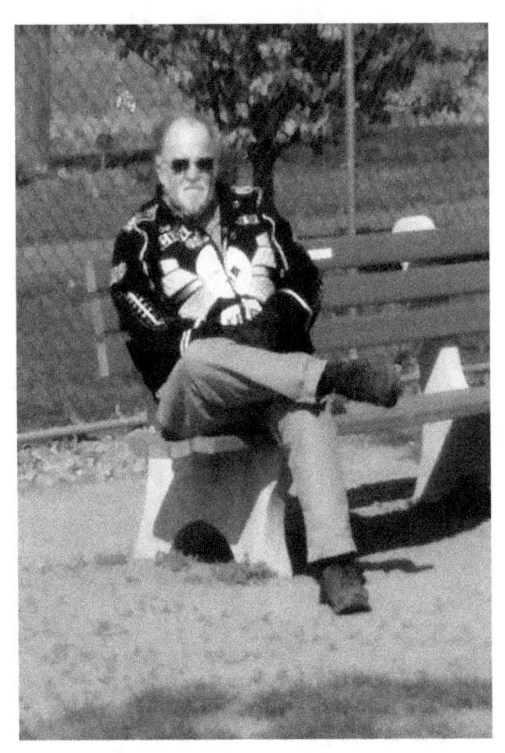

www.ingramcontent.com/pod-product-compliance
Lightning Source LLC
Chambersburg PA
CBHW071526180526
45171CB00002B/393